Healthy Healing Library Series
by
Linda Rector-Page, N.D., Ph.D.

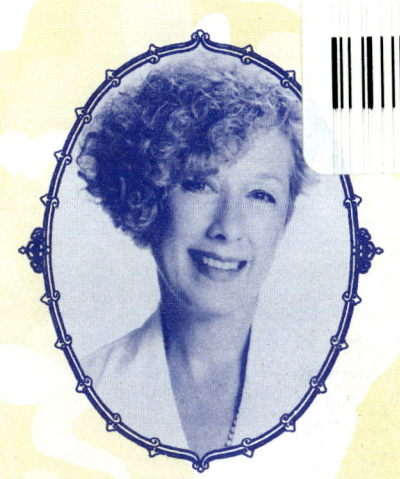

Allergy Control & Management

Fighting Asthma With Herbal Therapy

The Healthy Healing Library Series

As affordable health care in America becomes more difficult to finance and obtain, more attention is being focused on natural therapies and healthy preventive nutrition. Over 65% of Americans now use some form of alternative health care, from vitamins to massage therapy to herbal supplements. Everyone wants and needs more information about these methods in order to make informed choices for their own health and that of their families.

Herbal medicines are especially in the forefront of modern science today because they have the proven value of ancient wisdom and a safety record of centuries.

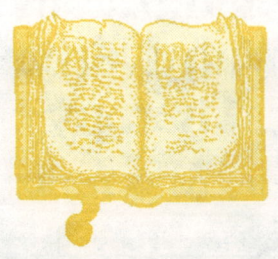

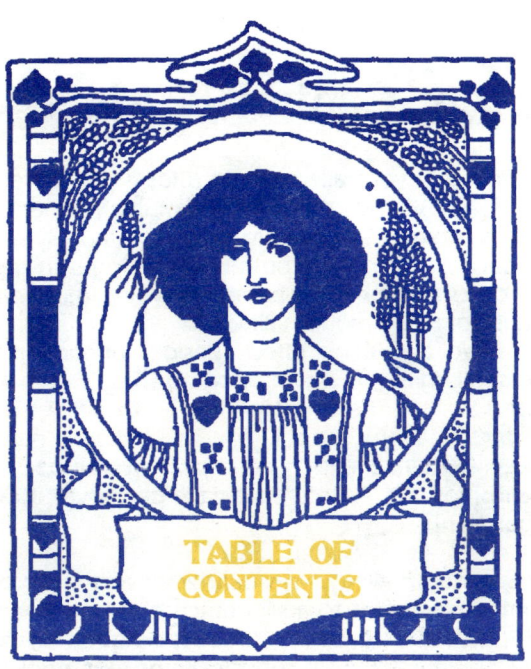

TABLE OF CONTENTS

* **All Types of Allergies are on the Rise** — **Pg. 5**

* **The Predominant Types of Allergens** — **Pg. 7**
  - Environmental & Seasonal Allergies — **Pg. 7**
  - Allergies to Chemicals & Contaminants — **Pg. 7**
  - Food Sensitivities & Intolerances — **Pg. 8**

* **Can Lifestyle Changes Help Prevent Allergic Reactions?** — **Pg. 10**

* **Is There Real Hope for Asthma Relief from Alternative Medicines?** — **Pg. 19**

* **Can Diet & Lifestyle Changes Help Prevent Asthma?** — **Pg. 21**
  - Mucous Cleansing Diets — **Pg. 21**
  - Herbal Remedies — **Pg. 22**
  - Effective Supplements — **Pg. 23**
  - Bodywork Techniques — **Pg. 23**

* **What About Childhood Asthma?** — **Pg. 24**

* **About Herbs & How They Work** — **Pg. 25**

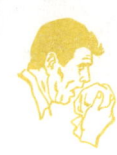

Allergy Control & Management

If it seems that your allergies are a lot worse in recent years, you may be right. Allergy reactions are multiplying across the board, manifesting themselves not only in the common symptoms of sneezing, headaches and rashes, but also as changes in personality, emotions, or one's sense of well-being. They are frequently an unrecognized cause of many modern illnesses.

Allergies have a domino effect. Besides uncomfortable, unsightly symptoms, allergies can be imprisoning. They can make it impossible to go for a walk in the country, or even to go outside for fresh air. They restrict healthful aerobic exercise because congested sinuses lead to less efficient breathing and poor overall body function. They limit friendships with friends that have pets (over 80% of the American population).

In times past, an allergy was defined as an inappropriate response by the immune system to a substance that is not normally harmful. While this definition is still true, there is no question that the harmful burden of inherently toxic substances on our bodies is increasing. Impaired immune response is one of the primary causes of allergies, especially when it becomes stressed by toxic overload. Negative factors like air, soil and water pollutants, acid rain, UV radiation caused by the depletion of the earth's protective ozone layer, chemically treated foods, compromised intestinal flora from over-reliance on antibiotics and steroid drugs, disturbance of infant immune systems through repeated vaccination and immunization, not to mention our stress-infused lifestyles, result in reduced immune response and the inability of our bodies to cope with or neutralize allergens.

The immune defense system is the most complex in the human body. Only recently are we beginning to understand its nature and comprehensive dynamics. It is a wonderful, autonomic, subconscious defense system that can hold off and neutralize pathogens so the body can heal itself. It is this quality of being a part of us, yet not under our conscious control, that is its greatest power. **And also its greatest problem.** When immune response is continually involved in fighting a "rear guard" action against a constant overload of immune-depressing, toxic substances, it gets to a point where it cannot distinguish harmful cells from healthy cells, and attacks everything. In many instances, if we can just "get out of the way" by limiting overkill from steroids and antibiotics, and keeping our bodies well-nourished and clear of toxic wastes, the immune system will function at its best.

Allergy Control & Management

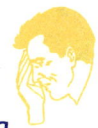

Immune response works by identifying foreign bodies and using the body's white blood cells to fight them. In some allergy reactions the immune system mis-identifies a substance as an invader, the white blood cells overreact and do more damage to the body than the invader. In other reactions to some of today's toxins, the immune system may overreact to the unknown, man-made chemical make-up in an effort to identify and overcome it. In either case, the allergic response becomes a disease in itself. Common responses are asthma, eczema, hayfever or severe headaches.

Research on the immune system shows that allergy-prone people produce an over-abundance of certain complex proteins known as antibodies. These in turn, trigger special cells known as mast cells that release inflammation-causing chemicals throughout the body. These chemicals, called histimines and leukotrienes, must either be neutralized by a severe allergic reaction or prevented from being released by an optimal lifestyle therapy program.

A strong immune system is critical for dealing with today's allergic reactions to pollutants; it is imperative in the prevention of modern opportunistic diseases such as herpes, lupus, candida albicans, or chronic fatigue syndrome that have allergic reactions as part of their symptomology.

The substances that cause allergies are called allergens. They can stem from any and all origins, but the most common allergens are grass pollen, dust, certain metals, some cosmetics, lanolin, hair and dander from some animals, insect bites or stings, some common drugs, some foods, and some additives and chemicals found in soaps. Most of these allergens produce clogging and congestion as the body tries to seal them off from its regular processes, or tries to work around them. Extra mucous is formed as a shield around the offending substances, and we get the allergy symptoms of sinus clog, stuffiness, hayfever, headaches and watery, puffy eyes. Sometimes the body tries to throw this excess off through the skin, and the irritation symptoms of rashes, fever blisters, abscesses or scratchy sore throat occurs. Allergies can affect any part of the body.

Drugs and over-the-counter medicines only relieve allergy symptoms. Cortisone, Prednisone, and similar steroid-type drugs taken over a long period of time for allergy symptoms do not cure, and often make the situation worse by depressing immune response and impeding elimination, harboring allergens inside the body. The natural healing way addresses the cause of the allergy to bring about more permanent improvement. This takes several months of time, and conscious effort and attention, but the rewards are worth it.

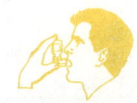

Allergy Control & Management

There are three broad categories of allergies:

❶ Allergies to environmental pollutants and seasonal conditions, called Type 1 allergies.

They exhibit symptoms called allergic rhinitis, symptoms we most associate with allergies, including hayfever's sinus congestion and itchy, watery nose and eyes, headaches, sneezing, coughing, scratchy throat, face swelling, insomnia, fatigue, skin itching and rashes.

Asthma is the most serious Type 1 allergy reaction.

The most common causes of environmental allergies stem from two main areas: 1) allergic reactions to air pollutants such as asbestos, heavy metals, smoke and fumes; 2) allergic reactions to seasonal factors such as dust, pollen, spores and molds.

This type of allergy often develops when the body has an excess accumulation of mucous that harbors the allergen irritants.

Common drugstore medications for environmental allergies only mask symptoms, often cause undesirable drowsiness, and also have a rebound effect. The more you use them the more you need them. Steroid compound drugs for environmental allergies, especially if taken over a long period of time, depress natural immune defenses and impede allergen irritant elimination.

In addition, allergens often interact in the systems of many allergy and asthma sufferers. Symptoms may be both activated and aggravated by a combination of offending irritants. When this is the case, even the most powerful drugs do not relieve the symptoms.

❷ Allergies to chemicals and contaminants, often designated Type 2 allergies.

Allergic reactions to chemicals are frequently a result of the body's attempt to isolate offending substances from its delicate balance and functions by storing them in fatty tissue. The allergic reaction occurs **after the second exposure to the irritant,** as the body's inflammatory response is alerted and histimines are produced. Repeated exposures to the irritant set off massive free radical reactions when the body's contaminate toleration levels are reached, toxic overload results and an allergic reaction set in.

Unfortunately, chemical hypersensitivity also initiates other forms of allergy, so that the sufferer becomes allergic to nearly everything else.

Chemical/contaminant allergies are characterized by migraine headaches, hyperactivity (especially in children), depression, anxiety, mood swings, personality changes, confusion and memory loss.

Allergy Control & Management

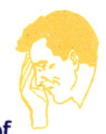

Common chemical/contaminant irritants vary, from a wide range of petro-chemicals to combustion residues from household appliances and heating systems, to various kinds of sprays, paints and exhaust fumes. Other culprits include chlorine bleach, moth balls and insect repellents, dry cleaning chemicals, and clothes that have been chemically treated.

❸ **Allergies, intolerances and sensitivities to certain foods or food additives, are also called Type 2 allergies.**

Food allergies are extremely widespread. Food sensitivities and intolerances are the fastest growing form of allergic reactions in the U.S. today, as more people are more and longer exposed to chemically altered, processed foods that the human body cannot handle. Essentially, a food allergy is an antibody response to a certain food. A food intolerance is an enzyme deficiency to digest a certain food. Both types of reactions can occur to either foods or food additives. Food sensitivities are similar to allergies in body reactions, but differ in that no antigen-specific antibodies are present in the sufferer. In general, they are not a permanent condition.

Food intolerances are often confused with food allergies. The estimated one in ten people with a lactose intolerance may experience the bloating, abdominal pain and diarrhea of an allergy reaction. But the symptoms are really due to a deficiency of the enzyme lactase, which breaks down milk sugar for proper digestion. A true food allergy involves immune system response when it encounters a food it views as a pathogen or parasite; a process, involving the food allergen itself, IgE antibodies, mast cells and basophils.

Common food intolerances include those to wheat, dairy products, fruits, sugar, yeast, mushrooms, eggs, coffee, corn and greens. Although these foods may be healthy in themselves, they are often heavily sprayed or treated, and in the case of animal products, also affected by anti-biotics and hormones.

Most food reaction symptoms are similar. Inflammation is generated by the release of histimines into the mast cells of the tissues, walling off the affected body area until immune response agents can restore health. But this process takes time. If the body is re-exposed before health is renewed, inflammation and consequent mucous congestion become chronic.

Food allergies may be hereditary, with a child being twice as likely to develop allergies if one parent has them, or four times as likely if both parents have them.

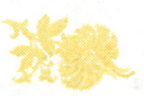
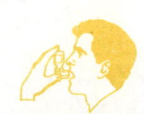

Allergy Control & Management

Conventional medical treatment for most allergies consists of antihistamines, steroids and desensitization shots. In obstinate cases, laser surgery may be used to vaporize mucus-forming nasal tissue. People with allergies know that these treatments do not work because they don't get to the cause of the problem. At best they provide temporary relief of symptoms; at worst, they create side effects which may be worse than the allergy itself.

Empowering your immune response is the key to overcoming allergies. Natural therapies are a much better choice for this effort because they are essentially immune enhancers working at the deepest levels of body functions. One of the greatest misunderstandings about allergies is the assumption that the allergen (the cat dander, the pollen, the house dust, etc.) is the problem. In reality the allergen is just the trigger, the allergic person is the loaded gun. Rather than just treating the symptoms or avoiding the allergen (which is never completely possible), the best course is to strengthen the body's immune defense system.

Research on the immune system shows that allergy-prone people produce an overabundance of certain complex proteins known as antibodies, which, in turn, trigger specialized cells known as mast cells, which then release chemicals that produce inflammation throughout the body. These chemicals, especially histamines and leukotrienes, must either be neutralized by a severe allergic reaction or prevented from being released by an optimal nutrition program.

The immune system is the body's most sensitive platform for nutritional support or for nutritional deficiency. Most disease environments are generated by lack of sufficient minerals and oxygen in the body's vital fluids, allowing pathogenic organisms to take hold. Normal immune response is reduced by the very things that cause allergies - air and water pollutants, toxic household substances, chemically treated foods, drugs, stress, and poor nutrition. Providing immune-enhancing nutrients at the first sign of infection or loss of health vastly improves the body's defense shield.

An effective, system strengthening formula for immunity might look like the one below. Most people experience improvement in 3 to 6 days. It may be used for continued results for 2 to 4 months.
Ingredients: The Food Blend: Miso Pwd., Soy Protein, Soy Sauce Pwd., Cranberry Pwd., Brewer's Yeast, Vegetable Acidophilus. **The Herbal Blend:** Alfalfa Lf., Borage Sd., Yellow Dock Rt., Oatstraw, Dandelion Lf., Barley Grass, Licorice Rt., Watercress Lf., Pau d'Arco Bk., Nettles Lf., Horsetail Herb, Red Raspberry Lf., Fennel Sd., Siberian Ginseng Rt., Parsley Rt. & Lf., Bilberry Bry., Schizandra Rt., Rosemary Lf. **The Sea Vegetable Blend:** Dulse, Wakame, Kombu, Sea Palm.

Allergy Control & Management

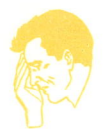

Can lifestyle changes help prevent allergies?
Diet change and herbal remedies are the most beneficial, quickest natural healing choices for overcoming and neutralizing allergens. Stress reduction techniques are pivotal, since stress and tension aggravate allergies. Exercise is also important to increase oxygen uptake in the lungs and tissues and to enhance immune response.

> Herbal combinations may be used to work with or follow a cleanse, or may be taken by themselves as tonics, to help neutralize allergens, increase oxygen uptake, stimulate adrenal activity, detoxify from pollutants, and allow work or sleep while you address the cause of the problem.

Every allergy type responds well to natural remedies. What are the primary lifestyle therapies to use in a program to overcome environmental allergies?

❦The best way to begin is often with a short three to seven day cleansing diet to rid the body of excess mucous build-up, and pave the way for diet and nutritional changes to have optimum effect. See "HEALTHY HEALING" or "COOKING FOR HEALTHY HEALING" by Linda Rector-Page for detailed examples of allergy detox diets.
After the cleansing, elimination diet, keep the body clear of congestion with non-mucous-forming foods such as fresh fruits and vegetables, whole grains, sea foods and cultured foods like yogurt. Avoid refined and preserved foods, dairy products and fatty, fried foods because they harbor congestive mucous pockets.

❦Herbal and homeopathic remedies are good choices as primary natural allergy medicines without side effects. They are specifics in addressing the following critical areas.

❦**Adrenal gland health** is fundamental in normalizing body functions against all kinds of allergies. Herbal compounds for adrenal support help stimulate and nourish exhausted adrenals, so that they can produce adrenal cortex and rebalance energy levels. Healthy adrenals are especially necessary in controlling environmental allergies. An effective herb capsule formula might look like this:
Ingredients: Licorice Rt., Sarsaparilla Rt., Bladderwrack, Uva Ursi, Rose Hips/vit. C, Irish Moss, Ginger Rt., Astragalus Rt., Capsicum, Pantothenic Acid 25mg, Vit. B6 20mg, Betaine HCL.

Allergy Control & Management

Men are particularly susceptible to adrenal fatigue. An effective herbal extract combination that seems to work particularly well for a man's system might look like this:
Ingredients: Licorice Rt., Sarsaparilla Rt., Bladderwrack, Irish Moss. Alcohol content 45%.

Some herbs work as natural antihistimines and decongestants for sinus and bronchial areas. The first capsule formula listed here helps keep passages open and offending allergens neutralized to avoid irritant build-up. It is most effective for hayfever and pollen allergies, often performing even when over-the-counter or prescription remedies have failed. Improvement may be noticed within an hour.
Ingredients: Marshmallow Rt., Burdock Rt., Mullein Lf., Goldenseal Rt., Parsley Rt., Acerola Cherry, Ma Huang Herb, Capsicum, Rosemary Lf., White Pine Bk., Pantothenic Acid 25mg.

The second capsule formula is largely symptomatic for relief of painful inflammation, sinus headaches, stuffiness and watery eyes. It may be used on an as-needed basis to let you work or sleep while your body is addressing the allergy cause.
Ingredients: Marshmallow Rt., Ma Huang Herb, Bee Pollen, White Pine Bk., Goldenseal Rt., Burdock Rt., Juniper Bry., Parsley Rt., Acerola Cherry, Rosemary Lf., Mullein Lf., Capsicum, Lobelia Lf., Pantothenic Acid 20mg., Vit B6 20mg.
Both formulas are fast acting, and work well on an as-needed basis for any allergy condition where these symptoms are present.

A natural antihistimine extract provides concentrated support for overcoming environmental allergens; it also encourages production of natural antihistimines by the body. It may be taken under the tongue on an as-needed basis during high risk seasons.
Ingredients: Ma Huang Herb, Mullein Lf., Marshmallow Rt., Goldenseal Rt., Burdock Rt., Wild Cherry Bk., Licorice Rt., Cinnamon Bk., Essential Oils Of Wintergreen & Lime. Alcohol Content 50%.

The following, gentle herb tea is a balancing compound that helps open clogged sinus and throat passages while alkalizing acid-producing allergens. The formula includes bee pollen making it quite effective against seasonal pollens and plant dusts in the air.
Ingredients: Horehound Lf., Peppermint Lf., Rose Hips, Ma Huang Herb, Rosebuds, Bee Pollen, Anise Sd., Ginger Rt., Orange Peel, Cloves, Burdock Rt.

➥The single herb, **GINKGO BILOBA**, taken several times daily as an extract is helpful in inactivating many biochemical allergens.

Allergy Control & Management

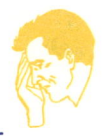

First line homeopathic remedies are renowned for their effectiveness against allergy reactions. Bioforce POLLINOSAN tablets is a good over all choice for many people. Homeopathic micro-doses of Allium Cepa, Nux Vomica, Eyebright and Pulsatilla are also effective when used for specific allergy symptoms. The best way to know which is right for you is to see a qualified homeopath.

❦Dietary supplements help reinforce the body's defenses against allergens and build body resistance to further attacks. Three products stand out from the rest for effective help:
❶ CO Q_{10} 60mg. - 3 to 4x daily.
❷ Quercetin - 2000mg. daily with Bromelain 500mg. daily.
❸ Ester C with bioflavonoids, up to 10,000mg. daily at first for detoxification, reducing to 3 to 5000mg. daily during allergy season.

❦Mild aerobic exercise, such as a daily brisk walk, is important for any program to overcome allergies. It increases oxygen uptake by the body, and enhances immune response by balancing body chemistry. If you need another reason to stop smoking, both smoking and secondary smoke magnifies allergy reactions.
❦Effective acupressure points for relief during an allergy attack are the tip of the nose and the hollow above the upper lip.

Chemical/contaminant irritants are complex and tough. Is a lifestyle therapy program effective in overcoming them?
The first concern in dealing with chemical contaminants should be eliminating from the body as quickly as possible. We find that a short liver-purifying cleanse is the most effective way to start. See "HEALTHY HEALING" or "COOKING FOR HEALTHY HEALING" by Linda Rector-Page for full details.

❦A diet improvement program against chemical allergies should also include a concentrated "green superfood" support and digestive support.
❶Since many chemical irritants can cause blood toxicity, we recommend a chlorophyll-rich green drink to balance and normalize the body. Many people don't realize that plant chlorophyllins are quite close in their structure to human plasma. A series of green drinks might be viewed as giving yourself a little "transfusion." An effective energizing green drink formula might look like this:
Ingredients: Rice Protein, Barley Grass, Apple Pectin, Alfalfa Lf., Bee Pollen, Siberian Ginseng Rt., Sarsaparilla Rt., Acerola Cherry, Chlorella, Dandelion Rt. & Lf., Dulse, Oats, Licorice Rt., Lemon Juice Pwd., Gotu Kola Lf.

Allergy Control & Management

❷Herbal bitters and green tea are the two natural therapy choices to enhance digestive efficiency. An effective green tea cleansing detox drink might look like this:
Ingredients: Bancha Lf., Burdock Rt., Kukicha Twig, Gotu Kola, Fo-ti Rt., Hawthorn Bry., Orange Peel & Oil, Cinnamon Bk. & Oil.

⮞Herbal bitters help insure good liver function, a key to the body's processing of chemical contaminants. Bitters are best taken in extract form in the morning.
Ingredients: Oregon Grape Rt., Gentian Rt., Cardamom Pods., Lemon Peel, Senna Lf., Dandelion Rt., Peppermint Lf., Honey. Alcohol Content 40%.

❸**Other important diet watchwords:** have a green salad every day, and take a glass of fresh carrot juice every other day for the first month of your program. On alternate days, have one to two cups of miso broth with dried, snipped sea vegetables on top, to enhance immune response and build potassium levels.

Herbal and homeopathic remedies for chemical allergies should concentrate on blood and liver cleansing as well as eliminating chemical and heavy metal residues from the body.
❶A gentle but effective way to start a liver cleanse might be with a liver flush tea like the one below to get your liver "liv-ing" again.
Ingredients: Dandelion Rt., Watercress Lf., Yellow Dock Rt., Hyssop Herb, Pau d'Arco Bk., Parsley Lf., Oregon Grape Rt., Red Sage & Oil, Licorice Rt., Milk Thistle Sd., Hibiscus Flr.
⮞The tea may be taken with the following capsule formula for stronger, broader cleansing effects.
Ingredients: Beet Rt., Oregon Grape Rt., Dandelion Rt., Wild Yam Rt., Milk Thistle Sd., Yellow Dock Rt., Ginkgo Biloba Lf., Wild Cherry Bk., Licorice Rt., Gotu Kola Lf., Ginger Rt., Barberry Bk., Choline 10mg, Inositol 10mg.

❷Certain herbs are specialized allergen neutralizers for those working around hazardous or toxic chemicals, or those sensitive to chemical air pollutants. These herbs help eliminate heavy metal residues from the body, and when taken with 5 to 10,000mg. of ascorbate vitamin C, help antioxidant activity and immune response.
Ingredients: Ascorbate Vit. C, Bladderwrack, Kelp, Bugleweed, Astragalus Rt., Prickly Ash Bk., Licorice Rt., Parsley Rt., Potassium (Chloride) 15mg.
⮞Grapefruit Seed Extract capsules have been an important addition in dealing with this type of allergy because they deal effectively with the inflammation and infection that often accompany it.

Allergy Control & Management

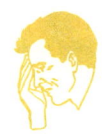

When considering dietary supplements for a chemical allergy program, I feel that antioxidants are by far the most important agents for dealing with exposure to toxins. Antioxidants should be in the diet supplement program for everyone today as a measure of protection against pollutants. In allergy-prone people, chemical exposures set off rampant free radical reactions, resulting in abnormal metabolism, altered protein synthesis, chronic inflammation and auto-immune antibodies such as those found in arthritis. If you choose a vitamin-type antioxidant supplement, choose one that includes raw glandulars and amino acids for best results.

Antioxidants from herbal sources combine directly with the body's own enzyme activity for enduring immune enhancement benefits.

☛An herbal capsule compound with antioxidant activity might look like this:
Ingredients: Rosemary Lf., Hawthorn Lf., Flr. & Bry., Siberian Ginseng Rt., Echinacea Purpurea Rt., Echinacea Angustifolia Rt., Pau d'Arco Bk., Milk Thistle Sd., Red Clover Blm., Licorice Rt., Astragalus Rt., Lemon Peel, Bilberry Lf. & Bry., Garlic, Ginkgo Biloba Lf., Spirulina, Capsicum, Ginger Rt.

Inflammation and low-grade infections in the head and chest are a trademark of chemical and contaminant allergies.
Herbs can be considered a specific to flush and clear the lymphatic system so that it can process infective toxins naturally out of the body, and relieve inflammation. These formulas are effective alone or used with other allergy fighting combinations to increase proficiency. Improvement is often noticed within a day.

☛A capsule combination with antibiotic activity looks like this:
INGREDIENTS: Echinacea Angustifolia Rt., Goldenseal Rt., Capsicum, Myrrh Gum, Yarrow Flr., Marshmallow Rt., Echinacea Purpurea Rt. & Lf., Black Walnut Hulls, Elecampane Rt., Turmeric Rt., Potassium Chloride 15mg.

☛An equally effective extract combination that works to reduce inflammation looks like this:
INGREDIENTS: Echinacea Angustifolia and Purpurea Rt., Lf. & Flr., Goldenseal Rt., Pau d'Arco Bk., Myrrh Gum, Vegetable Glycerine, Wintergreen Oil. Alcohol content 55%.

Note: Avoid the use of commercial antacids if possible. They interfere with enzyme production and the ability of the body to eliminate chemical residues.

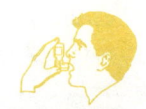

Allergy Control & Management

It has been said that any one at any time can be allergic to almost any food. Can lifestyle therapy help seemingly random food allergies?

Food allergy reactions appear most often in hyperactive children, in young adults, and more often in men than women. The most common determinant of food allergies is thought to be incomplete digestion, caused by enzymatic imbalances that show up as a low grade inflammation of the bowel lining. Since many children that have allergies grow out of them, it is thought that these enzyme imbalances normalize as their immune and digestive systems mature.

The obvious way to avoid a food allergen is to eliminate it. Repeatedly ingesting foods that cause allergy reactions intensifies allergy symptoms, because more and more antibodies are released to fight them. Unfortunately, in an allergy prone person, the most frequently eaten foods seem to be the allergy source and the cause of immune system problems. Reactions can range from mild hives to full-blown anaphylactic shock.

There are three self-diagnostic tests allergy sufferers can use to detect their food allergy without painful skin scratch tests.

❶ The first is an elimination diet. Eliminate common allergy foods until symptoms lessen; then re-introduce the foods to see which ones cause the symptoms to return. Re-introduction should be done slowly and carefully to avoid severe reactions. Some allergens are very potent. People who react strongly to nuts may experience anaphylactic shock just eating from a bowl that contains traces of nuts. Elimination diet techniques have had success in that a third of food allergy sufferers grow out of their allergy after a year or two of elimination.

❷ The second is a rotation diet. To detect the allergen food, eat only a single food at a meal for four days. Then don't eat it again for four days. Re-introduce the food on the fifth day. If a flare-up occurs, one is allergic to that food. Most people need to repeat this rotation plan on a variety of foods to really understand their allergies.

❸ The third is the Coca Pulse Test, named after Arthur Coca, founder of the Journal of Immunology. Dr. Coca discovered that eating allergy-producing foods causes a big increase in the heart beat, often 20 or more beats above average. If you suspect a food allergy but have not yet determined which food, Dr. Coca's self diagnosis test may help. The test is as follows: take your resting pulse upon rising. Then, eating only one food at a time, take your pulse reading five, 30 and 60 minutes after eating that food. If your pulse rises more than 20 beats a minute on any of these measurements, eliminate that food for at least 30 days. Reintroduce it gradually to see if it produces any allergy symptoms.

Allergy Control & Management

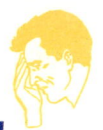

A comprehensive, natural therapy program for getting rid of food allergies might include:

🌀Diet techniques to help your digestion as well as to reduce food sensitivity, because good digestion will lessen the burden of antigens in the digestive tract.

- Make good food-combining a part of your eating habits. (See "COOKING FOR HEALTHY HEALING" for a complete discussion of food combining.)
- Improve your bowel health with a high-fiber, low-fat diet.
- Foods to include in your diet should be cultured foods like yogurt and kefir to add friendly flora to the digestive tract, plenty of green, leafy vegetables (high in fiber and magnesium), orange and yellow vegetables (high in fiber and beta carotene), and fresh fruits (high in fiber, vitamin C and bioflavonoids). New research shows that a naturally occurring compound in fresh fruits and vegetables minimizes allergy responses.

🌀Dietary supplements that can help restore your immune system:

❶ The bioflavonoid quercetin has powerful antioxidant effects and decreases inflammation damage by inhibiting histimine release.

❷ Vitamin C with bioflavonoids, another powerful antioxidant that acts as a natural antihistimine and is essential for proper adrenal gland function; take up to 5000mg. daily.

❸ CoQ10, 60mg. twice daily to help the liver produce antihistimines.

❹ Vitamins A and zinc to help correct leaky gut syndrome.

❺ Omega-3 fatty acids to reduce allergic reactions by inhibiting leukotriene and prostaglandin inflammation.

🌀Herbal therapy for food allergies is a two-pronged protocol.

- Herbs are superb at helping the body normalize antihistimine production against allergy reactions because they work at the deepest levels of the body processes. A capsule combination to help cleanse and stimulate the liver in this effort might look like this:
Ingredients: Beet Rt., Oregon Grape Rt., Dandelion Rt., Wild Yam Rt., Milk Thistle Sd., Yellow Dock Rt., Ginkgo Biloba Lf., Wild Cherry Bk., Licorice Rt., Gotu Kola Lf., Ginger Rt., Barberry Bk., Choline 10mg, Inositol 10mg.

- Enzyme activity is the key to understanding food allergy reactions. Herbal plant enzymes often work when antacids or even commercial enzyme products do not, because they are naturally-occurring, highly complex in the broad range of their activity, yet easily assimilated by the body to help digestion and improve tolerance of food allergens.

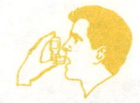

Allergy Control & Management

Two formulas in particular are recommended for allergy sufferers.
◖The first is an herbal bitters compound to help the production of bile for more complete digestion.
Ingredients: Oregon Grape Rt., Gentian Rt., Cardamom Pods., Lemon Peel, Senna Lf., Dandelion Rt., Peppermint Lf., Honey. Alcohol Content 40%.
◖The second is a pre-meal enzyme formula with a long history of success against a wide range of allergy/related digestive problems.
Ingredients: Fresh Ginger Rt., Peppermint Lf., Fennel Sd., Catnip Herb, Cramp Bark, Spearmint Lf., Turmeric Rt., Papaya Lf. Alcohol Content 45%.

⚜

There are three allergy-related areas where herbal therapy can be of great help.
❦Candida albicans yeast overgrowth, a plaguing, auto-immune imbalance of modern civilization is always characterized by allergy reactions to a wide range of foods and contaminants. Naturopaths today, also recognize "leaky gut syndrome" as an allergy response of candida. Leaky gut is a condition of the intestinal tract where large molecules, particularly proteins, pass through the gut membranes into the blood stream and become irritants or antigens. They are intercepted by the immune system and dealt with in several ways. The body may attempt to engulf and destroy them through inflammatory allergy responses; or it may deposit the substances in various tissues resulting in kidney problems or joint pain.

Herbal treatments as part of a candida healing program have had notable success. They are a gentle, long lasting remedies to help correct body imbalances and enhance immune response. There are usually multiple allergies in conjunction with a candida infection. Best results are obtained if they are treated systemically, both to curtail the infection and to reculture the colon. A broad spectrum formula to help kill the yeasts and restore normalize intestinal function might look like this:
Ingredients: Pau d'Arco Bk., Vegetable Acidophilus, Black Walnut Hulls, Garlic, Barberry Bk., Sodium Caprylate, Spirulina, Rose Hips/Vit. C, Cranberry Pwd., Licorice Rt., Burdock Rt., Echinacea Angustifolia Rt., Echinacea Purpurea Rt., Peppermint Lf., Thyme Lf., Rosemary Lf., Dong Quai Rt., Damiana Lf., DL-phenylalanine 10mg, Zinc (Gluconate) 3mg, Calcium (Citrate) 3mg.
◖Take with quercetin with bromelain 1000 to 2000mg. daily.
◖Take with garlic capsules, 6 to 10 daily.
◖Take with **BLACK WALNUT EXTRACT** and/or **ASHWAGANDHA EXTRACT** as specifics for immune enhancement.

Allergy Control & Management

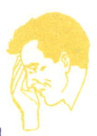

☙Take with the following tea, 2 to 3 cups daily for extra gland balance and lymphatic cleansing.
Ingredients: Pau d'Arco Bk., Cranberry Pwd., Rose Hips, Damiana Lf., Burdock Rt., Echinacea Purpurea Rt., Myrrh Gum, Lemon Balm Lf., Cinnamon Bk. & Oil, Hibiscus Flowers.

Herbal combinations are effective in relieving the skin itching and scaling common to food or chemical allergies. As most allergy sufferers know, the skin is one of the primary outlets for a histimine reaction in the form of red bumps, rashes and painful hives. Certain herbs can help neutralize these irritant acid wastes that the body is throwing off through the skin. The following formula is effective both internally and externally; simply soak cotton balls in the strained tea and apply to rashes or irritation.
Ingredients: Burdock Rt., Licorice Rt., St. John's Wort Lf., Dandelion Rt., Yellow Dock Rt., Borage Sd., Chamomile Flr., Red Clover Blm., White Sage Lf. & Oil, Calendula Flr.

The most overlooked characteristic in treating allergic conditions, is the presence of chronic fungal and parasitic infections. Nearly all persons afflicted with allergic disorders display one or both of these conditions. Health experts estimate that over half of the American population will, at some point become host to some kind of parasite. Both fungal and parasitic organisms excrete toxic wastes into the tissues, causing tissue damage and inflammation, and reducing immune response. Both set up allergic reactions through this tissue damage, by impairing digestion because food is not broken down completely and by damaging the intestinal villi. Partially digested macro-molecules of food are then absorbed through the damaged intestinal walls and released as inflammatory products that circulate, irritating tissues, and causing allergic reactions. Parasites are a major factor in damaging the intestinal walls and should be considered early in any type of allergy treatment program, because tissues are unlikely to heal while these organisms thrive.
The following herbal compound has been used for decades as an effective vermifuge for parasitic infective organisms.
Ingredients: Black Walnut Hulls, Garlic, Pumpkin Sd., Gentian Rt., Butternut Bk., Fennel Sd., Cascara Sagrada Bk., Mugwort Lf., Slippery Elm Bk., False Unicorn Rt.

Getting allergies out of your life will lift an unpleasant burden you have probably been living with for years.

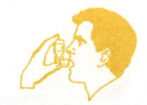

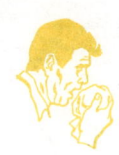

Allergy Control & Management

Overcoming Asthma

Asthma is a life-threatening allergic reaction, but until recently was considered to be a mild condition that one got over or grew out of. However, new statistics show that 12 million Americans (and perhaps many more undiagnosed) currently have asthma, compared to 6.8 million in 1980, an increase of 30% in the last decade alone. U.S. hospital admission rates due to asthma have almost quadrupled in the last two decades and reported deaths due to asthma have jumped 68% in the same period. Hospitalization cost for asthma treatment in 1993 was over 6.5 billion! Mortality rates due to asthma have increased more than 30%. This same severe trend is being experienced in almost every industrialized nation. Traditional medicine has no cure.

Asthma affects certain groups of people more than others. More children are affected by asthma than adults; it is the most frequent cause of missed school. Even if a child grows out of severe attacks he or she remains at risk. New studies show that the underlying inflammation of asthma never goes away. More males get asthma with a 2:1 ratio of boys to girls; blacks are slightly more likely to have asthma than whites but are twice as likely to die from it. The greatest increase in asthma deaths has occurred in people 65 years old and over.

While new gene research seems to indicate hereditary pathways, naturopaths believe that an increasingly polluted environment is partially to blame for asthma attacks. They also see our "prescription-happy" society as a reason for the increase in asthma, because strong drugs in general suppress the immune system, and asthma is one of a long list of immune deficient conditions that are common in modern developed countries. Traditional medicine is also coming to the conclusion that using inappropriate asthma drugs may be playing a role in the upswing of attacks and especially of deaths due to attacks. A recent study in the New England Journal of Medicine showed that heavy use of a common broncho-dilator called a beta-agonist correlated with an increased risk of death from asthma. Other research suggests that certain synthetic broncholdilators also increase the asthma death rate. Asthmatics who turn frequently to bronchodilators may actually need anti-inflammatory drugs instead.

Before an asthma attack, inflammation of the lining of the bronchial tubes causes them to swell and steps up production of thick, sticky mucus that further reduces the narrow tubes. The inflamed

Allergy Control & Management

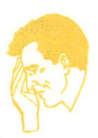

airways become very unstable meaning that the slightest provocation can lead to an asthma attack.

While there is no question that asthmatic attacks are triggered, the triggers are quite different for different people. Triggers are as diverse as allergens like air pollutants, pollens, perfumes, animal fur or feathers, cold, dry air, cigarette smoke, dusts, chemicals such as solvents and paints, emotional stress or upset, or even a viral cold or flu. The food allergy/asthma link is well-known, including dairy products and eggs, and especially triggers from foods containing monosodium glutamate (MSG) and sulfiting agents used widely in wine, beer, and snacks. Certain medications, including aspirin can also provoke asthma. The most common circumstance under which asthma develops is just from lying down; it's the reason doctors tell patients to sleep with their head and shoulders elevated.

Many asthmatics have found that alternative therapies enable them to cut back, even in some cases eliminate, their need for conventional, drug-dependent treatment. Because of their nature, quitting asthma drugs too quickly can bring on an attack, but we heartily recommend working with a physician who also uses alternative therapies, or one who supports your efforts to reduce asthma drugs while using alternative treatments.

An effective program using alternative therapies and techniques would include four main areas of treatment.

❶ A mucous cleansing liquid diet, followed by a non-mucous-forming maintenance diet and elimination of food allergens.
❷ Herbal remedies that help reduce inflammation, encourage antihistimine production, gently dilate bronchial airways, relax involuntary spasms, support adrenal gland function, and allow more tissue oxygen uptake through antioxidant activity.
❸ A supplement program that includes powerful antioxidants, Omega-3 fatty acids, and pantothenic acid therapy within the B Complex vitamin spectrum.
❹ Bodywork that may include acupuncture, deep breathing exercises, an herb-infused vaporizer at night, stress-reduction techniques, such as biofeedback or meditation, and hydrotherapy.

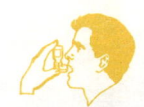

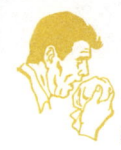

Allergy Control & Management

✌A mucous cleansing diet helps both allergies and asthma:

Diet and nutritional improvement should clearly be part of a program to overcome asthma permanently. In our experience, this always involves avoiding refined sugars, pasteurized dairy, and/or wheat products. Even when these foods are not direct asthma provocations they alter the body's acid/alkaline balance and increase the production of mucous. Other substances to avoid should include alcohol, caffeine, additives, colorings and non-food chemical irritants.

Any program to overcome asthma or allergies will benefit from a short mucous elimination diet. This allows the body to rid itself of toxins and mucous accumulations before an attempt to change eating habits. The first vitamin C rich stage is summarized below. It should be followed for 3 to 5 days. It often produces symptomatic relief from asthma in 24 to 48 hours.

On rising: take a glass of cranberry, apple or grapefruit juice; **or** lemon juice in hot water with 1 teasp. honey; **or** a glass of cider vinegar, hot water and ginger syrup.

Breakfast: take a Knudsen's VERY VEGGIE JUICE with 1 teasp. liquid chlorophyll, or 1 teasp. BRAGG'S LIQUID AMINOS, and/or 1 TB. olive oil added. **Add** 2 or 3 garlic capsules and 1/4 to 1/2 teasp. ascorbate vitamin C or Ester C powder with bioflavonoids in water.

Mid-morning: have a glass of fresh carrot juice; **and/or** a cup of of any of the herb teas listed on the next page.

Lunch: have a hot vegetable, miso or onion broth. **Add** 2 to 3 more garlic capsules and 1/4 to 1/2 teasp. ascorbate vitamin C or Ester C powder with bioflavonoids in water.

Mid-afternoon: have a cleansing herb tea, such as alfalfa/mint.

Dinner: have a hot veggie broth, another glass of Knudsen's VERY VEGGIE JUICE, or miso soup with dried sea veggies snipped on top; **or** another glass of carrot juice with 1 TB. olive oil added. Take 2 to 3 more garlic capsules, and 1/4 to 1/2 teasp. ascorbate vitamin C or Ester C powder in water.

Before bed: take another hot water, lemon and honey drink; **or** hot apple or cranberry juice with ginger syrup.

Note #1: Drink six to eight glasses of bottled water or mineral water each day for best cleansing results.

Note #2: Add 1 teasp. acidophilus liquid, or 1/4 to 1/2 teasp. acidophilus pdr. to any broth or juice to balance the digestive system.

Note #3: Any of the therapeutic herb teas listed on the next page may be taken during the mucous cleansing diet for increased results.

Allergy Control & Management

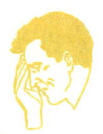

A vegetarian diet provides significant improvement in asthma cases, because it eliminates most common food allergens and favorably alters fatty acid metabolism. Ninety-two percent of the patients who completed one study reported improvement in their asthma, as well as a reduction of infectious diseases. Seventy-one percent of the patients responded within four months; one year of the vegetarian diet was required before the 92 percent level was reached.

For a long term maintenance diet, avoid pasteurized dairy products, heavy starches and refined foods that are inherently a breeding ground for continued congestion.
Eat foods high in omega-3 fatty acids, such as salmon or tuna and plenty of fruits and vegetables. Emphasize complex carbohydrates that are high in fiber, such as whole grains, beans, and vegetables, and reduce intake of animal fats, fried foods, alcohol and simple sugars (most asthmatics also suffer from hypoglycemia).

❧Herbal teas to include in a mucous cleanse:
A balancing, cleansing and stimulating tea with antioxidants:
Ingredients: Bancha Lf., Burdock Rt., Kukicha Twig, Gotu Kola Lf., Fo-ti Rt., Hawthorn Bry., Orange Peel & Oil, Cinnamon Bk.

A broncho-dilating tea to open breathing airways and soothe irritated membranes, with expectorant herbs to clear mucous congestion.
Ingredients: Marshmallow Rt., Fenugreek Sd., Mullein Lf., Ma Huang Herb, Wild Cherry Bk., Ginkgo Biloba Lf., Rosemary Lf., Angelica Rt., Passionflowers, Cinnamon Bk., Lobelia Lf.

A tea to address deep-seated, deep lung congestion.
Ingredients: Wild Cherry Bk., Mullein Lf., Safflowers, Ma Huang Herb, Sage Lf., Ginger Rt., Pleurisy Rt., Thyme Lf., Blackberry Lf., Parsley Lf., Lobelia Lf.

A tea to encourage better oxygen uptake by the body
Ingredients: Fenugreek Sd., Hyssop Herb, Horehound, Ginkgo Biloba Lf., Rose Hips, Ma Huang Herb, Marshmallow Rt., Boneset Lf., Anise Sd., Peppermint Lf., Wild Cherry Bk., Lobelia Lf.

❧Supplements to help overcome asthma:
❶ Antioxidants in the form of vitamin C or Ester C with bioflavonoids, 3000 to 5,000mg. daily, and/or Quercetin 1000 to 2000mg. daily with bromelain for uptake, 500mg. daily.
❷ Omega-3 fatty acids in the form of fish or flax oil, or essential fatty acids such as Evening Primrose oil, 1000mg. daily.

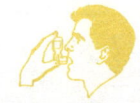

Allergy Control & Management

❸B Complex 100mg. daily with extra pantothenic acid, 1000mg. daily, extra B12, 2500mcg. daily, and extra B6 100mg. daily.
❹Shark oil extract, a fatty acid that reduces the body's inflammatory response to PAF's (platelet-activating-factors), that often trigger allergies and asthma. Take 750mg., 1 to 2 daily.

Note: Try to stay away from cortisone compounds that eventually weaken the immune system, and from over-the-counter drugs that often simply drive the congestion deeper into the lungs and tissues.

❦The complexity of advanced herbal compounds is a good approach for the complexity of asthma's causes and symptoms, without the side-effects engendered by drug treatments.

Herbs have a long history of being able to help asthmatics, because their broad spectrum, yet specific activity can address so many symptoms of asthma.

- They can help reduce painful inflammation:
Ingredients: White Willow Bk., St. John's Wort Lf., Echinacea Angustifolia Rt., Echinacea Purpurea Rt., White Pine Bk., Gotu Kola Lf., Red Clover Blsm., Devil's Claw Rt., Alfalfa Lf. Pwd., Bromelain 22mg, Burdock Rt., Dandelion Rt., Chamomile Flr., Uva Ursi Lf., Ginger Rt.

- They can help calm and control choking, and wheezing caused by the extreme difficulty of exhalation during an asthmatic attack. They may be used, 4 at a time as needed, to help relieve involuntary constriction and contraction of the respiratory muscles.
Ingredients: Cramp Bark, Black Haw Bk., Rosemary Lf., Kava Kava Rt., Passionflower Flr., Red Raspberry Lf., Wild Yam Rt., St. John's Wort Lf., Chaste Tree Bry., Kelp, Lobelia Lf., Valerian Rt.

- They can increase and support oxygen uptake in the respiratory system while strengthening lung, respiratory and circulatory functions. A strong nervine is included in the following formula for antispasmodic activity, with vitamin C herbs to encourage antihistimine activity and antioxidant herbs for immune enhancement.
Ingredients: Bee Pollen, Bupleurum Rt., White Pine Bk., Elecampane, Royal Jelly, Scullcap Lf., Ma Huang Herb, Acerola Cherry, Ginger Rt.

- They may be used on a regular basis to control chronic body stress and tension, or as needed to help quiet the spasms of an acute asthmatic attacks. The following formula is a strong nervine and muscle relaxant, that works quite rapidly in this regard, often when nothing else is effective.

Allergy Control & Management

Ingredients: Ashwagandha Rt. & Lf., Black Cohosh Rt., Scullcap Lf., Kava Kava Rt., Black Haw Bk., Hops, Valerian Rt., European Mistletoe, Wood Betony Lf., Lobelia Lf., Oatstraw.

- Asthmatic stress impairs adrenal function in varying degrees, which then becomes a co-factor in the glandular imbalances of asthma. The following herbal compounds help stimulate and nourish exhausted adrenals, so that they can produce adrenal cortex and re-balance energy levels. Healthy adrenal activity is beneficial for many asthmatic syndromes, from sinus clog to hypoglycemic reactions. The first is a capsule formula:

Ingredients: Licorice Rt., Sarsaparilla Rt., Bladderwrack, Uva Ursi, Rose Hips/vit. C, Irish Moss, Ginger Rt., Astragalus Rt., Capsicum, Pantothenic Acid 25mg, Vit. B6 20mg, Betaine Hcl.

The second is an extract formula:

Ingredients: Licorice Rt., Sarsaparilla Rt., Bladderwrack, Irish Moss. Alcohol Content 45%.

☙Effective single herbs might include GINKGO BILOBA EXTRACT, a PAF inhibitor to reduce inflammation, and known allergy triggers.

☙A synergistic compound of LICORICE ROOT and GINSENG ROOT combines the well-known antiinflammatory, anti-allergy activity of licorice root with the adaptogenic, tissue-tonifying qualities of PANAX GINSENG.

☙What are some natural bodywork techniques that may reduce asthma attacks?

❶**Acupuncture, biofeedback and reflexology** methods have all shown good results for asthma.

❷**Meditation and stress-reduction techniques** such as a weekly massage therapy treatment are beneficial.

❸**Fresh air exercise** and deep diaphragmatic breathing are keys to permanent success over asthma, to increase regular oxygen uptake, and to keep body passages open.

❹**Hydrotherapy** in the form of hot fomentations to the chest, may help during an acute attack. Combine the compresses with hot foot baths, keeping the head cool with cool compresses, and the body covered up with cotton blankets.

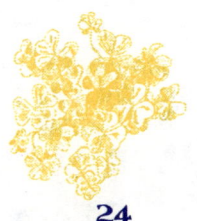

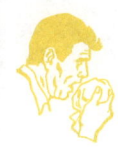

Allergy Control & Management

What About Childhood Asthma?

Asthma is getting deadlier for children. Recent studies show that mortality among children under 15 is doubling every ten years. Until recently, childhood asthma was considered a psychosomatic illness, an overreaction to stress, or a bid for attention. Today, experts believe the alarming increase in air pollution contaminants affects a child's small airway passages even worse than an adult's. They see children as more susceptible to asthma because they have smaller lungs and bronchial tubes, and less breathng reserve when under attack by allergies or breath-sapping pollutants. In addition, they are more susceptible to colds, a major trigger for asthma attacks. Naturopaths believe childhood asthma is related to too-early weaning (before the first birthday), and an early introduction of too many wheat and pasteurized dairy foods. Dairy products, are widely recognized as problem foods for many asthmatic children.

A child developing asthma exhibits several early symtoms. First, colds are never simple and are often accompanied by ear infections, a harsh cough that sounds like a seal barking, and wheezing. In an asthmatic child, wheezing is a tight, dry sound like a high whistle. Wheezing is most common at night and often accompanied by a dry cough. More than one or two such episodes in a season is usually diagnosed as asthma.

Some children outgrow asthma; this is most likely if asthma attacks are kept to a minimum in the first place through carefully managed diet, exercise and a lot of love and affection.
The following herbal formulas are especially gentle, yet effective for childhood asthma. The other herbal compounds detailed in this booklet are also effective for children with appropriate dilutions. (See page 28 for child doses.)

➧The herbal compound below acts as an expectorant to release mucous buildup in the head and chest. It is reliable for children where a mild but effective remedy is required on an as-needed basis. Effects are quickly noticeable.
Ingredients: Ma Huang Herb, Licorice Rt., Mullein Lf., Rose Hips, Marshmallow Rt., Peppermint Lf., Fennel Sd., Boneset Lf., Ginger Rt., Calendula Flr.

➧A **VALERIAN/WILD LETTUCE EXTRACT** may also be used as a spasm control and relief during attack. It may be taken in water or under the tongue, is safe for children, and is especially useful at night when coughing and choking prevent sleep and rest.
Ingredients: Valerian Rt., 50%, Wild Lettuce Leaf, 50%.

Allergy Control & Management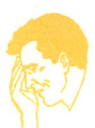

About Herbs and How They Work

What are herbs?

Herbs are concentrated foods, edible plants that are safe to take as foods, but are also rich in nutrients that can stimulate the body's healing force, and balance and regulate the human system.

1) Herbs can nourish us, especially with minerals, bolstering deficiencies from poor soil and environment.

2) Herbs can stimulate the body's healing processes by working with the system as body balancers.

Herbal combinations are not addictive or habit-forming, but they are powerful nutritional agents that should be used with common sense and care. Balance is the key to using herbal nutrients for healing. It takes a little more attention and personal responsibility than mindlessly taking a prescription drug. The results are worth it for long term health.

Even though herbs are concentrated, they are whole - not partitioned or isolated substances like drugs. Many drugs use plant isolates and concentrates, but herbs are not drugs. When dealing with chronic long standing problems, I believe the value of herbs lies in their wholeness, not in their concentration. You should not expect the same kind of activity or response that you experience from a chemically formed compound. Drugs treat the symptoms of a problem, so you generally have to take more and more of a drug to get the same effect. It is usually wise to take herbs in descending strength, asking your body to pick up more of its own work.

How do herbs work?

Herbs are foundation support nutrients, working through the glands, nourishing the body's deep-seated elements, such as the brain and the endocrine system. Results will seem to take longer. This is because herbs are working at the deepest levels of body balance and chemistry. **They work at the cause of the problem.** The effects are much more permanent.

Yet, even with slow steady action, most people feel improvement from herbal treatment in three to six days. Chronic, long standing problems will take longer. The standard rule of thumb is one month of healing for every year of the problem.

Herbs do not work like drugs or even like vitamins, where excess amounts flush through the body. Herbs work through the body's enzyme activity, combining with you in the same way that food does. (You are what you eat.) Herbs also contain food enzymes themselves. Their nutritional elements accumulate in the body.

I am always being asked to formulate an herbal maintenance multiple, but I don't think this would serve people well. Taking the same herbs all the time would be like eating the same foods all the time. It would lead to imbalanced nutrition from nutrients that were not in those foods.

Allergy Control & Management

Multiple vitamins also work best when strengthening a weak or deficient system. They are not a substitute for a balanced diet.

Herbs work better in combination than they do singly. There are several reasons for this.

1) Each compound contains two to five primary agent herbs that are part of the blend for specific purposes. Since all body parts, and most disease symptoms, are interrelated, it is wise to have herbs which can affect each part of the problem.

2) Body balance is encouraged by a combination of herbal nutrients, rather than a large supply of one or two focused properties. A combination gently stimulates the body as a whole.

3) A combination allows inclusion of herbs that work at different stages of need.

4) A combination of several herbs with similar properties can increase the latitude of effectiveness, not only through a wider range of activity, but also reinforcing herbs that were picked too late or too early, or grew in adverse weather conditions.

5) No two people, or their bodies, are alike. Good response is better insured by a combination of herbs.

6) Finally, some very potent and complex herbs, such as capsicum, lobelia, sassafras, mandrake, tansy, canada snake root, wormwood, woodruff, poke root, and rue are beneficial in small amounts and as catalysts, but should not be used alone.

➥For more information, see "HOW TO BE YOUR OWN HERBAL PHARMACIST," a book that clearly shows people how to make and use herbal compounds for themselves, rather than to just use single herbs.

What might I experience during herbal therapy?

1) Occasionally you might experience a mild allergy type reaction as might occur in response to a food. In almost every case, this is not due to the herb itself, but to the chemicals or pesticides used in the growing or storing process; or because incompatible herbs might have been used together; or just an individual adverse reaction. The key to avoiding adverse reactions is moderation. Anything taken to excess can cause a negative side effect. Use common sense when taking herbs as foods or medicines.

2) As with other natural healing programs, you may experience a healing crisis during herbal treatment. This is the "law of cure" and simply means that you seem to get worse before you get better, as the body goes through a cleansing process to eliminate toxins. Most of us recognize this as the headache, slight nausea and weakness we feel during a cleansing fast. If there is too much discomfort, simply pace back the herbal treatment to a more comfortable level, and let it take a little longer.

How can I take herbs safely for the best results?

1) Herbs are plants for problems. They work best when used on an as-needed basis. **Herbal formulas can be quite specific for a need. Take the formula for your condition at the right time, not all the time, or best results.**

Allergy Control & Management

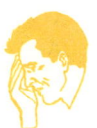

Also, rotating and alternating herbal combinations according to your health goals will allow the body to remain most responsive to their effects.

> **Like the rest of the natural universe, herbs seem to work better with the body when taken for six days in a row, with a rest on the seventh day.**

2) Take herbs in descending strength, resting on the seventh day each week. Start with greater amounts at the beginning of your program to build a good healing base. As you observe your health returning, fewer and fewer of the large initial doses should be taken. At the end of the program you should be taking maintenance dosage for prevention. **For most people, they realize an herbal treatment has done its job when they forget to take it.**

3) It is better to take only one or two herbal combinations at the same time. Choose the treatment that addresses your worst problem first. One of the bonuses of a natural healing program is the discovery that other problems were really complications of the worst one. They will often take care of themselves.

4) Give herbs time to work. Especially with severe, immune deficient, degenerative diseases, it takes a great deal of time to rebuild health. Patience is not an American virtue, but it is important not to add more, except under a qualified practitioner's care, even when your program is working and you are improving. We find that trying to speed up benefits often only aggravates symptoms and brings worse results. **Moderate amounts are excellent, mega-doses are not.** This is because the immune system is a very fragile entity, and can be overwhelmed instead of stimulated. A strong, virulent virus can even be nourished and mutate through supplementation instead of arrested by it. Give yourself more time and gentler treatment. Like most other things in life, it ain't just what you do, it's also the way that you do it.

5) Herbs should not be taken like vitamins, i.e. as maintenance to shore up nutrient deficiencies. Except for some food grown vitamins, vitamins are partitioned substances. They don't combine with the body the way herbs do. Excesses are normally flushed through the system if they are not needed. Herbs combine with the body through it's enzyme activity.

Are herbs safe for children?

Herbs are generally very safe for children. Herb dosage for children (and adults) should be based on body weight:
Child dosage is as follows:
1/2 dose for children 10-14 years
1/3 dose for children 6-10 years
1/4 dose for children 2-6 years
1/8 dose for infants and babies

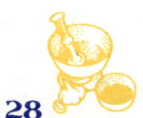

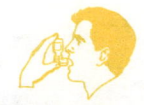

The effective lifestyle therapy programs offered in this booklet have been developed over the last fifteen years from the reported responses and successful healing results experienced by literally thousands of people. In addition, the full time research team at Healthy Healing Publications investigates herbs, herbal combinations and herbal therapies from around the world for their availability and efficacy. You can feel every confidence that the recommendations are synthesized from real people with real problems who got real results.

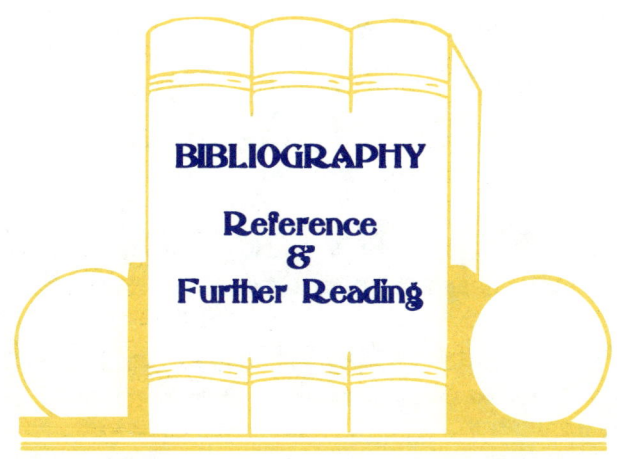

BIBLIOGRAPHY
Reference & Further Reading

Balch, James F., M.D., and Balch, Phyllis A., C.N.C. **Prescription for Healthy Healing.** Garden City Park, New York: Avery Publishing Group Inc., 1990.

Bland, Jeffery, Ph.D. "The Key to the Power of Vitamin C and its Metabolites," **Self-Care Health Library**. New Canaan, Conn.: Keats Publishing, Inc., 1989.

Braly, James, M.D. **Food Allergy and Nutrition Revolution**. New Cannan, Connecticut: Keats Publishing, 1992.

Firshein, Richard. "Treating Asthma Without Drugs." **Natural Health**, July/August 1994.

Hobbs, Christopher. "The Contemporary Herbal: Herbs For Hay Fever." **Total Health**, June 1992.

Hoffman, David. **The Herbal Handbook**. Rochester, Vermont: Healing Arts Press, 1988.

Holmes, Peter. **The Energetics of Western Herbs Vol. I & II**. Berkeley: NatTrop Publishing, 1993.

Levin, Alan, and Zellerbach, Maria. **Type1, Type 2 Allergy Program**. Los Angeles: Jeremy Tarcher, 1983.

Lichtenstein, Lawerence M. "Allergy and the Immune System." **Scientific American**, Sept., 1993.

Mowery, Daniel B., Ph.D. **Herbal Tonic Therapies**. New Canaan, Conn.: Keats Publishing, Inc., 1993.

Mowery, Daniel B., Ph.D **The Scientific Validation of Herbal Medicine**. New Canaan, Connecticut: Keats Pub. 1986.

Neuchard, Ellen, and Feinstein, Alice. **Fighting Disease: The Complete Guide to Natural Immune Power**. Emmaus, Pa.: Rodale Press, 1989.

Pendersen, Mark. **Nutritional Herbology Vol. I & II**. Bountiful, Utah: Pendersen Publishing, 1991.

Quillin, Patrick. **Healing Nutrients**. Chicago: Contemp. Bks, 1987.

Weiner, Michael A., Ph.D. **Maximum Immunity**. New York: Pocket Books, 1987.

Weiner, Michael A., Ph.D., and Weiner, Janet A. **Herbs that Heal.** Mill Valley, California: Quantum Books, 1994.

Zand, Janet, LAc, OMD. **Smart Medicine For A Healthier Child**. Garden City, New York: Avery Publishing Group, 1994.

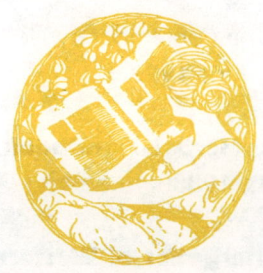

Dr. Page's written papers are thoroughly researched - through empirical observation as well as from internationally documented evidence. Studies are ongoing and updated. If you desire reference material, send a self-addressed, stamped envelope with your request to Healthy Healing Publications, 16060 Via Este, Sonora, Ca., 95370.

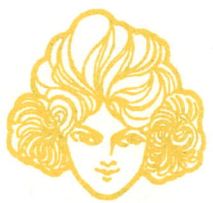

Booklets in the Library Series

- Renewing Female Balance
- Do You Have Blood Sugar Blues?
- A Fighting Chance For Weight Loss & Cellulite Control
- The Energy Crunch & You
- Gland & Organ Health - Taking Care
- Heart & Circulation - Controlling Blood Cholesterol
- Detoxification & Body Cleansing to Fight Disease
- Allergy Control & Management; Fighting Asthma
- Stress Management, Depression; Addictions
- Colds & Flu & You - Building Optimum Immunity
- Fighting Infections with Herbs - Controlling STDs
- Beautiful Skin, Hair & Nails Naturally
- Don't Let Your Food Go to Waste
- Do You Want to Have a Baby? Natural Prenatal Care
- Menopause & Osteoporosis
- Power Plants - Boosting Immunity With Herbs
- Herbal Therapy For Kids
- Renewing Male Health & Energy
- Cancer - Can Alternative Therapies Help?
- "Civilization" Diseases - CFS, Candida, Lupus & More
- Overcoming Arthritis With Natural Therapies

Dr. Page's written papers are thoroughly researched - through empirical observation as well as from internationally documented evidence. Studies are ongoing and updated. If you desire reference material, send a self-addressed, stamped envelope with your request to Healthy Healing Publications, 16060 Via Este, Sonora, Ca., 95370.

ABOUT THE AUTHOR

Linda Rector-Page has been working in the fields of nutrition and herbal medicine both professionally and as a personal lifestyle choice, since the early seventies. She is a certified Doctor of Naturopathy and Ph.D., with extensive experience in formulating and testing herbal combinations. She received a Doctorate of Naturopathy from the Clayton School of Holistic Healing in 1988, and a Ph.D. in Nutritional Therapy from the American Holistic College of Nutrition in 1989. She is a member of both the American and California Naturopathic Medical Associations.

Linda opened and operated the "Rainbow Kitchen", a natural foods restaurant, then became a working partner in The Country Store Natural Foods store. She has written four successful books and a library series of booklets in the nutritional healing field. She is the founder/developer of Crystal Star Herbal Nutrition.

Broad, continuous research in all aspects of the alternative healing world, from manufacturers, to stores to consumers has been the cornerstone of success for her reference work **"HEALTHY HEALING,"** now in its ninth edition. Crystal Star Herbal Nutrition products, which are formulated by Linda, are carried by over twenty-five hundred natural food stores nationwide. Feedback from these consumer sources provides up-to-the-minute contact with the needs and results experienced by people taking more responsibility for their own health. Much of the lifestyle information and empirical observation in her books comes from this direct experience - knowledge that is then translated into Crystal Star Herbal Nutrition products, and recorded in every **"HEALTHY HEALING"** edition.

"COOKING FOR HEALTHY HEALING," now in its second new edition, is a companion to **"HEALTHY HEALING."** It draws on both the recipes from the Rainbow Kitchen and the defined, lifestyle diets that she has developed from healing results since then. The book contains 33 separate diet programs, and over 900 healthy recipes. Every recipe has been taste-tested and time-tested as part of each recommended diet so that the healing suggestions can be easily maintained with optimum nutrition.

In **"HOW TO BE YOUR OWN HERBAL PHARMACIST,"** Linda addresses the rising appeal of herbs and herbal healing in America. Many people are taking an interest in clearly understanding herbal formulation knowledge for personal use. This book is designed for those wishing to take more definitive responsibility for their health through individually developed herbal combinations.

Linda's newest work is a party reference book called **"PARTY LIGHTS"** in collaboration with restaurateur Doug Vanderberg. **"PARTY LIGHTS"** takes healthy cooking one step further by adding in the fun to a good diet. Over sixty party themes are completely planned in this new book, all with healthy party foods, earthwise decorations, professional garnishing tips, festive napkin folding, interesting games and activities.

Published by Healthy Healing Publications, 1995.